THE AUTOIMMUNE STANDARD LIFESTYLE DIET

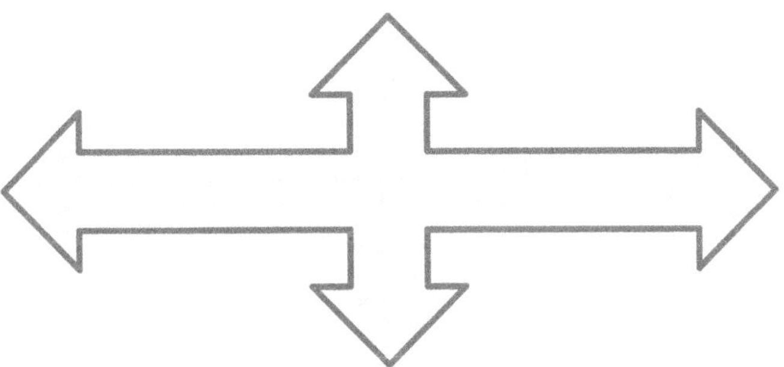

Nourishing Recipes: Embrace Optimal Health with The Autoimmune Standard Lifestyle Diet For overall wellbeing

DR.D.JOHNSTON

CONTENT

INTRODUCTION

Understanding Autoimmune Diseases

Autoimmune diseases occur when the body's immune system mistakenly attacks its own tissues, leading to inflammation, pain, and failure in different organs and systems. There are over 80 known autoimmune diseases, including rheumatoid arthritis, lupus, multiple sclerosis, and celiac disease. While the exact causes of autoimmune illnesses are not fully known, genetic susceptibility, external factors, and dysregulation of the immune system are thought to play important roles.

Overview of the Autoimmune Standard Lifestyle Diet

The Autoimmune Protocol (AIP) diet, also known as the Autoimmune Standard Lifestyle (ASL) diet, is a treatment method meant to lower inflammation and support healing in people with autoimmune illnesses. It includes removing foods that are known to cause immune reactions or add to inflammation, such as wheat, dairy, beans, nightshade veggies, processed foods, and refined sugars. Instead, the diet focuses on nutrient-dense whole foods that support gut health, lower inflammation, and provide important vitamins and minerals.

How This Cookbook Can Help

This guide is a valuable resource for people following the Autoimmune Standard Lifestyle (ASL) diet, giving a diverse array of delicious and healthy meals that fit with the principles of the plan. By offering innovative and flavorful recipes made from healthy ingredients, this guide makes it easier for individuals with autoimmune diseases to stick to their dietary rules while still having filling meals.

Each recipe in this guide is thoughtfully created to exclude common trigger foods and stress nutrient-rich ingredients that support general health and well-being. From breakfasts and snacks to main dishes and sweets, there are options for every meal and event, ensuring that people following the ASL diet never feel cheated or limited in their food choices.

In addition to giving delicious recipes, this guide also provides useful information on ingredient swaps, meal planning tips, and strategies for handling social settings while sticking to the ASL diet. By providing people with autoimmune diseases with useful tools and resources, this recipe serves as a helpful partner on their road to better health and energy.

In conclusion, this cookbook is more than just a collection of recipes—it is a complete guide to living well with inflammatory diseases. By adopting the principles of the Autoimmune Standard Lifestyle diet and adding healthy, delicious meals into their daily routine, people can take positive steps towards controlling their condition, lowering inflammation, and improving their overall quality of life.

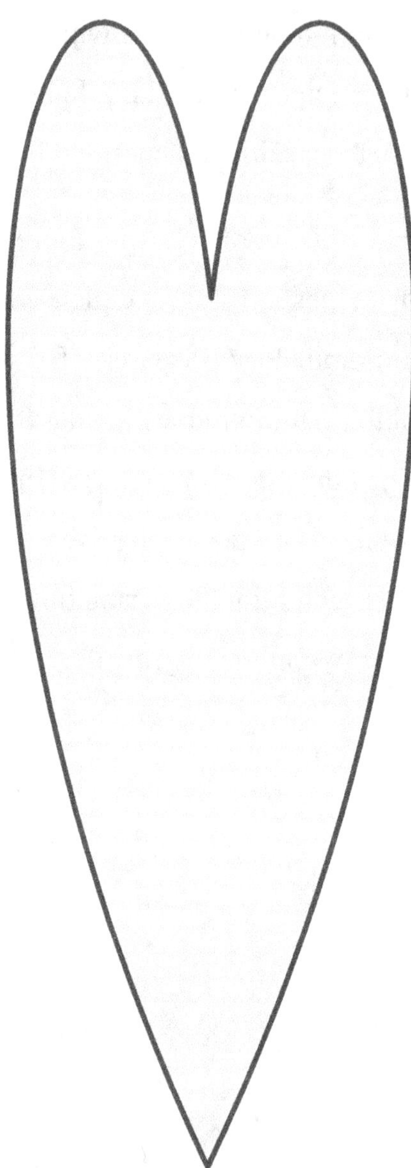

Chapter 1:

Getting Started

Assessing Your Current Diet and Lifestyle

Before starting on any dietary changes, it's important to review your present diet and lifestyle to spot areas for growth and possible causes for inflammatory symptoms. Keep a food log to track what you eat and how you feel afterward, marking any signs or responses you experience. Pay attention to trends and connections between certain foods and flare-ups of symptoms. Additionally, consider other living factors such as stress levels, sleep quality, exercise habits, and exposure to outdoor chemicals, as these can all impact autoimmune health.

Preparing Your Kitchen for Success

Setting up your kitchen for success is important when following the Autoimmune Standard Lifestyle (ASL) plan. Start by clearing out any processed foods, refined sugars, grains, dairy products, and other inflammatory ingredients from your pantry and refrigerator. Stock up on nutrient-dense whole foods such as fresh fruits and veggies, lean meats, healthy fats, herbs, and spices. Invest in cooking tools and equipment that make meal preparation faster, such as a mixer, food processor, quality knives, and storage bins for leftovers. Having a well-organized and stocked kitchen will make it easier to stick to your food goals and prepare healthy meals at home.

Shopping List Essentials

When making your shopping plan for the ASL diet, focus on buying a range of nutrient-dense whole foods that support gut health, lower inflammation, and provide important vitamins and minerals. Some shopping list basics include:

Fresh fruits and vegetables (especially leafy greens, spicy veggies, and bright nuts)

Lean meats (such as wild-caught fish, organic chicken, grass-fed beef, and pastured eggs)

Healthy fats (such as avocado, olive oil, coconut oil, and nuts/seeds)

Gluten-free grains (such as quinoa, rice, and gluten-free oats)

Herbs and spices (such as turmeric, ginger, garlic, and cinnamon)

Bone soup or collagen peptides for gut repair

Fermented foods (such as cabbage, kimchi, and coconut yogurt) for probiotics

Non-dairy milk options (such as almond milk or coconut milk)

Natural sweets (such as raw honey or maple syrup)

Meal Planning Tips

Meal planning is key to staying on track with the ASL diet and ensuring that you have healthy meals available throughout the week. Start by making a weekly meal plan that includes a range of recipes and tastes to keep meals interesting and enjoyable. Batch cook items such as meats, grains, and veggies ahead of time to save time during the week. Use leftovers artistically by adding them into salads, soups, or stir-fries. Experiment with different cooking methods and taste combinations to keep meals interesting. And don't forget to include plenty of snacks and easy grab-and-go choices for busy days.

By reviewing your current diet and lifestyle, setting your kitchen for success, stocking up on basics, and adopting effective meal planning methods, you can set yourself up for success on the Autoimmune Standard Lifestyle (ASL) diet. With commitment, stability, and a little imagination, you can enjoy delicious, healthy meals that support your autoimmune health and general well-being.

Chapter 2:

Breakfast

Morning Fuel: Breakfast Basics

Simple Avocado Toast

- o **Ingredients:**

    - 2 slices of gluten-free bread

    - 1 ripe avocado

    - Pinch of salt and black pepper

    - Optional toppings: sliced tomatoes, microgreens, hemp seeds

- o **Instructions:**

1. Toast the bread slices until golden brown.

2. Mash the avocado in a bowl and season with salt and pepper.

3. Spread the mashed avocado evenly onto the toast.

4. Top with desired toppings and serve immediately.

- o **Nutritional Value (per serving):**

  - Calories: 250 kcal

  - Protein: 5g

  - Carbohydrates: 25g

  - Fat: 15g

- o **Time per Serving**: 5 minutes

2. Nutrient-Dense Smoothies

Green Goddess Smoothie

- o **Ingredients:**

  - 1 cup spinach leaves

  - 1/2 ripe banana

  - 1/2 cup frozen pineapple chunks

  - 1/2 cup coconut water

- 1 tablespoon chia seeds

- Optional: 1 scoop of protein powder

- **Instructions:**

1. Add all ingredients to a blender.

2. Blend until smooth and creamy.

3. Pour into a glass and enjoy immediately.

- **Nutritional Value (per serving):**

- Calories: 180 kcal

- Protein: 5g

- Carbohydrates: 30g

- Fat: 6g

- **Time per Serving:** 5 minutes

3. Grain-Free Porridges and Cereals

Coconut Chia Seed Pudding

- **Ingredients:**

  - 1/4 cup chia seeds

  - 1 cup coconut milk

  - 1/2 teaspoon vanilla extract

  - Optional toppings: fresh berries, sliced almonds, shredded coconut

- **Instructions:**

1. In a bowl, combine chia seeds, coconut milk, and vanilla extract.

2. Stir well to combine and let sit for 5 minutes.

3. Stir again to break up any clumps and cover the bowl with plastic wrap.

4. Refrigerate overnight or for at least 4 hours until thickened.

5. Serve chilled with your favorite toppings.

- **Nutritional Value (per serving):**

- Calories: 220 kcal

- Protein: 5g

- Carbohydrates: 15g

- Fat: 15g

- **Time per Serving:** 10 minutes prep + overnight chilling

4. Protein-Packed Egg Dishes

Vegetable Egg Muffins

- **Ingredients:**

  - 6 eggs

  - 1/4 cup diced bell peppers

  - 1/4 cup diced onions

  - 1/4 cup chopped spinach

  - Salt and pepper to taste

  - Optional: grated cheese

- **Instructions:**

1.   Preheat the oven to 350°F (175°C) and grease a muffin tin.

2.   In a bowl, whisk together eggs, bell peppers, onions, spinach, salt, and pepper.

3.   Pour the egg mixture evenly into the muffin cups, filling each about 3/4 full.

4.   Bake for 20-25 minutes or until the eggs are set and slightly golden.

5.   Allow to cool slightly before removing from the muffin tin. Serve warm.

- **Nutritional Value (per serving):**

  - Calories: 150 kcal

  - Protein: 12g

  - Carbohydrates: 3g

  - Fat: 10g

- Time per Serving: 30 minutes

5. Creative Breakfast Bowls

Acai Berry Bowl

- o **Ingredients:**

    - 1 packet frozen acai puree

    - 1/2 cup frozen mixed berries

    - 1/2 banana, sliced

    - 1/4 cup granola

    - Optional toppings: sliced almonds, shredded coconut, honey

- o **Instructions:**

1. In a blender, combine frozen acai puree, mixed berries, and half of the sliced banana.

2. Blend until smooth and creamy, adding a splash of coconut water if needed.

3. Pour the smoothie into a bowl and top with granola, remaining banana slices, and desired toppings.

4. Serve immediately and enjoy!

- **Nutritional Value (per serving):**

  - Calories: 300 kcal

  - Protein: 5g

  - Carbohydrates: 45g

  - Fat: 12g

- **Time per Serving**: 10 minutes

Chapter 3:

Lunch

Simple Salad Creations

Mediterranean Chickpea Salad

- o **Ingredients:**

  - 1 can chickpeas, rinsed and drained

  - 1 cucumber, diced

  - 1 cup cherry tomatoes, halved

  - 1/4 cup red onion, thinly sliced

  - 1/4 cup Kalamata olives, pitted and sliced

  - 1/4 cup feta cheese, crumbled (optional)

  - 2 tablespoons extra virgin olive oil

  - 1 tablespoon lemon juice

- 1 teaspoon dried oregano

- Salt and pepper to taste

- **Instructions:**

1. In a large bowl, combine chickpeas, cucumber, tomatoes, red onion, and olives.

2. In a small bowl, whisk together olive oil, lemon juice, dried oregano, salt, and pepper.

3. Pour the dressing over the salad and toss to coat.

4. Sprinkle with crumbled feta cheese if desired.

5. Serve chilled and enjoy!

- **Nutritional Value (per serving):**

- Calories: 250 kcal

- Protein: 8g

- Carbohydrates: 30g

- Fat: 12g

- **Time per Serving: 15 minutes**

2. Nourishing Soups and Stews

Hearty Vegetable Quinoa Soup

- **Ingredients:**

  - 1 tablespoon olive oil

  - 1 onion, diced

  - 2 carrots, diced

  - 2 celery stalks, diced

  - 2 cloves garlic, minced

  - 1 teaspoon dried thyme

  - 1/2 teaspoon dried rosemary

  - 1/2 cup quinoa, rinsed

  - 4 cups vegetable broth

  - 1 can diced tomatoes

  - 2 cups chopped kale or spinach

  - Salt and pepper to taste

- **Instructions:**

1. In a large pot, heat olive oil over medium heat. Add onion, carrots, and celery, and cook until softened.

2. Add garlic, thyme, and rosemary, and cook for another minute until fragrant.

3. Stir in quinoa, vegetable broth, and diced tomatoes. Bring to a boil, then reduce heat and simmer for 15 minutes.

4. Add chopped kale or spinach and simmer for an additional 5 minutes until greens are wilted.

5. Season with salt and pepper to taste.

6. Serve hot and enjoy!

- **Nutritional Value (per serving):**
  - Calories: 200 kcal
  - Protein: 6g
  - Carbohydrates: 30g
  - Fat: 6g
- **Time per Serving: 30 minutes**

3. Wholesome Sandwiches and Wraps

Turkey and Avocado Wrap

- **Ingredients:**

  - 1 whole wheat or gluten-free wrap

  - 3 slices turkey breast

  - 1/4 avocado, sliced

  - Handful of mixed greens

  - 1 tablespoon hummus

  - 1 teaspoon Dijon mustard

- **Instructions:**

1. Lay the wrap flat and spread hummus and Dijon mustard evenly over the surface.

2. Layer turkey slices, avocado slices, and mixed greens on top of the wrap.

3. Roll up the wrap tightly, folding in the sides as you go.

4. Slice in half diagonally and serve immediately.

- o **Nutritional Value (per serving):**

  - Calories: 300 kcal

  - Protein: 20g

  - Carbohydrates: 30g

  - Fat: 12g

- o **Time per Serving: 10 minutes**

---

4. Energizing Buddha Bowls

Rainbow Buddha Bowl

- o **Ingredients:**

  - 1 cup cooked quinoa or brown rice

  - 1/2 cup cooked chickpeas

  - 1/2 cup shredded carrots

  - 1/2 cup sliced cucumber

  - 1/2 cup cherry tomatoes, halved

  - 1/2 avocado, sliced

  - Handful of mixed greens

- Tahini dressing (optional)

o **Instructions:**

1. In a bowl, arrange cooked quinoa or brown rice, cooked chickpeas, shredded carrots, sliced cucumber, cherry tomatoes, avocado slices, and mixed greens.

2. Drizzle with tahini dressing if desired.

3. Serve immediately and enjoy!

o **Nutritional Value (per serving):**

- Calories: 350 kcal

- Protein: 12g

- Carbohydrates: 45g

- Fat: 15g

o **Time per Serving: 15 minutes**

5. Quick and Easy Lunchbox Ideas

Mason Jar Salad

- **Ingredients:**

  - 1 pint-sized mason jar

  - 2 tablespoons balsamic vinaigrette dressing

  - 1/2 cup cooked quinoa

  - 1/4 cup cherry tomatoes, halved

  - 1/4 cup diced cucumber

  - 1/4 cup shredded carrots

  - Handful of mixed greens

  - Optional toppings: cooked chicken breast, sliced almonds, feta cheese

- **Instructions:**

1. Pour balsamic vinaigrette dressing into the bottom of the mason jar.

2.   Layer quinoa, cherry tomatoes, cucumber, shredded carrots, mixed greens, and any optional toppings in the jar.

3.   Seal the jar tightly and refrigerate until ready to eat.

4.   Shake the jar before serving to distribute the dressing.

- **Nutritional Value (per serving):**

  - Calories: 250 kcal

  - Protein: 8g

  - Carbohydrates: 30g

  - Fat: 10g

- **Time per Serving: 10 minutes**

Chapter 4:

Dinner

1. Satisfying One-Pot Meals

Quinoa Vegetable Stir-Fry

- o **Ingredients**:

  - 1 cup quinoa, rinsed

  - 2 cups vegetable broth

  - 1 tablespoon sesame oil

  - 2 cloves garlic, minced

  - 1 tablespoon grated ginger

  - 1 cup sliced bell peppers

  - 1 cup broccoli florets

  - 1 cup sliced carrots

  - 1/2 cup snap peas

  - 1/4 cup soy sauce or tamari

  - 2 green onions, chopped

- Sesame seeds for garnish

  o **Instructions:**

1. In a large skillet or pot, heat sesame oil over medium heat. Add minced garlic and grated ginger, and sauté for 1 minute.

2. Add quinoa and vegetable broth to the skillet. Bring to a boil, then reduce heat, cover, and simmer for 15 minutes.

3. Stir in sliced bell peppers, broccoli florets, sliced carrots, and snap peas. Cook for an additional 5-7 minutes until vegetables are tender.

4. Stir in soy sauce or tamari and chopped green onions.

5. Garnish with sesame seeds before serving.

  o **Nutritional Value (per serving):**

- Calories: 300 kcal

- Protein: 10g

- Carbohydrates: 45g

- Fat: 8g

- ○ Time per Serving: 30 minutes

---

2. Flavorful Stir-Fries and Skillets

Ginger Garlic Chicken Stir-Fry

- ○ **Ingredients:**

    - ▪ 1 lb chicken breast, thinly sliced

    - ▪ 2 tablespoons soy sauce or tamari

    - ▪ 1 tablespoon rice vinegar

    - ▪ 1 tablespoon sesame oil

    - ▪ 2 cloves garlic, minced

    - ▪ 1 tablespoon grated ginger

    - ▪ 2 cups mixed vegetables (bell peppers, broccoli, carrots, snap peas)

    - ▪ Cooked rice or cauliflower rice for serving

    - ▪ Green onions and sesame seeds for garnish

- ○ **Instructions:**

1. In a bowl, marinate sliced chicken breast in soy sauce or tamari, rice vinegar, and sesame oil for 15 minutes.

2. Heat a large skillet or wok over medium-high heat. Add marinated chicken and cook until browned and cooked through, about 5-7 minutes.

3. Add minced garlic and grated ginger to the skillet and cook for another minute until fragrant.

4. Add mixed vegetables to the skillet and stir-fry until tender-crisp, about 3-5 minutes.

5. Serve stir-fry over cooked rice or cauliflower rice, garnished with chopped green onions and sesame seeds.

- **Nutritional Value (per serving):**
  - Calories: 350 kcal
  - Protein: 30g
  - Carbohydrates: 20g
  - Fat: 15g
- Time per Serving: 30 minutes

Spinach and Mushroom Quinoa Casserole

- o **Ingredients:**

  - 1 cup quinoa, rinsed

  - 2 cups vegetable broth

  - 1 tablespoon olive oil

  - 1 onion, diced

  - 2 cloves garlic, minced

  - 8 oz mushrooms, sliced

  - 4 cups fresh spinach

  - 1/2 cup grated Parmesan cheese (optional)

  - Salt and pepper to taste

- o **Instructions:**

1. Preheat the oven to 375°F (190°C).

2.   In a large skillet, heat olive oil over medium heat. Add diced onion and minced garlic, and sauté until softened.

3.   Add sliced mushrooms to the skillet and cook until browned and tender.

4.   Stir in fresh spinach and cook until wilted.

5.   In a separate pot, cook quinoa according to package instructions, using vegetable broth instead of water.

6.   Combine cooked quinoa with the mushroom and spinach mixture. Season with salt and pepper to taste.

7.   Transfer the mixture to a baking dish and sprinkle with grated Parmesan cheese if desired.

8.   Bake in the preheated oven for 20-25 minutes until bubbly and golden brown.

- o **Nutritional Value (per serving):**
  - Calories: 250 kcal

- Protein: 12g

- Carbohydrates: 30g

- Fat: 10g

- **Time per Serving: 45 minutes**

4. Hearty Grain-Free Pastas

Zucchini Noodles with Pesto and Cherry Tomatoes

- **Ingredients:**

  - 2 large zucchinis, spiralized into noodles

  - 1 cup cherry tomatoes, halved

  - 1/4 cup homemade or store-bought pesto sauce

  - 1 tablespoon olive oil

  - Salt and pepper to taste

  - Optional: grated Parmesan cheese for serving

- **Instructions:**

1.   Heat olive oil in a large skillet over medium heat. Add spiralized zucchini noodles and cherry tomatoes.

2.   Cook for 3-5 minutes until zucchini noodles are tender-crisp and tomatoes are slightly softened.

3.   Stir in pesto sauce and toss until evenly coated.

4.   Season with salt and pepper to taste.

5.   Serve immediately, garnished with grated Parmesan cheese if desired.

- **Nutritional Value (per serving):**

  - Calories: 200 kcal

  - Protein: 5g

  - Carbohydrates: 10g

  - Fat: 15g

- Time per Serving: 15 minutes

5. Savory Roasts and Grilled Delights

Lemon Herb Grilled Chicken

- **Ingredients:**

  - 4 boneless, skinless chicken breasts

  - 2 tablespoons olive oil

  - Zest and juice of 1 lemon

  - 2 cloves garlic, minced

  - 1 teaspoon dried thyme

  - 1 teaspoon dried rosemary

  - Salt and pepper to taste

- **Instructions:**

1. In a bowl, whisk together olive oil, lemon zest, lemon juice, minced garlic, dried thyme, dried rosemary, salt, and pepper.

2. Place chicken breasts in a shallow dish or resealable plastic bag. Pour marinade over the chicken and toss to coat.

3. Cover and refrigerate for at least 30 minutes, or up to 4 hours.

4.   Preheat grill to medium-high heat. Remove chicken from marinade and discard excess marinade.

5.   Grill chicken for 6-8 minutes per side, or until cooked through and no longer pink in the center.

6.   Serve grilled chicken hot with your favorite side dishes.

- **Nutritional Value (per serving):**

  - Calories: 250 kcal

  - Protein: 30g

  - Carbohydrates: 1g

  - Fat: 12g

- **Time per Serving: 30 minutes**

Chapter 5:

Sides and Snacks

Crispy Veggie Chips and Dips

Baked Sweet Potato Chips

- o **Ingredients:**

  - 2 large sweet potatoes, thinly sliced

  - 2 tablespoons olive oil

  - Salt and pepper to taste

- o **Instructions:**

1. Preheat the oven to 375°F (190°C) and line a baking sheet with parchment paper.

2. In a bowl, toss sweet potato slices with olive oil, salt, and pepper until evenly coated.

3. Arrange sweet potato slices in a single layer on the prepared baking sheet.

4. Bake for 15-20 minutes, flipping halfway through, until crispy and golden brown.

5. Serve hot with your favorite dip.

Creamy Avocado Dip

- o **Ingredients:**

    - 2 ripe avocados

    - 1/4 cup Greek yogurt or dairy-free yogurt

    - Juice of 1 lime

    - 2 cloves garlic, minced

    - Salt and pepper to taste

- o **Instructions**:

    0. In a bowl, mash avocados until smooth and creamy.

    1. Stir in Greek yogurt, lime juice, minced garlic, salt, and pepper until well combined.

    2. Adjust seasoning to taste.

    3. Serve chilled with baked sweet potato chips or vegetable crudites.

Roasted Garlic Parmesan Broccoli

- o **Ingredients:**

  - 4 cups broccoli florets

  - 2 tablespoons olive oil

  - 2 cloves garlic, minced

  - 1/4 cup grated Parmesan cheese

  - Salt and pepper to taste

- o **Instructions:**

1. Preheat the oven to 400°F (200°C) and line a baking sheet with parchment paper.

2. In a bowl, toss broccoli florets with olive oil, minced garlic, grated Parmesan cheese, salt, and pepper until evenly coated.

3. Spread broccoli florets in a single layer on the prepared baking sheet.

4. Roast in the preheated oven for 15-20 minutes, until broccoli is tender and lightly browned.

5. Serve hot as a nutritious side dish.

3. Guilt-Free Snack Recipes

Spicy Roasted Chickpeas

- **Ingredients:**

  - 1 can chickpeas, rinsed and drained

  - 1 tablespoon olive oil

  - 1 teaspoon paprika

  - 1/2 teaspoon cayenne pepper

  - 1/2 teaspoon garlic powder

  - Salt to taste

- **Instructions:**

1. Preheat the oven to 400°F (200°C) and line a baking sheet with parchment paper.

2. Pat dry chickpeas with a paper towel to remove excess moisture.

3. In a bowl, toss chickpeas with olive oil, paprika, cayenne pepper, garlic powder, and salt until evenly coated.

4. Spread chickpeas in a single layer on the prepared baking sheet.

5. Roast in the preheated oven for 25-30 minutes, shaking the pan halfway through, until chickpeas are crispy.

6. Let cool before serving as a crunchy and spicy snack.

4. Fermented Foods for Gut Health

Homemade Sauerkraut

- o **Ingredients:**

  - 1 small head of cabbage, thinly sliced

  - 1 tablespoon sea salt

  - Caraway seeds (optional)

  - Filtered water

- o **Instructions:**

1.   In a large bowl, massage thinly sliced cabbage with sea salt until it starts to release its liquid.

2.   Add caraway seeds if desired for flavor.

3.   Pack the cabbage mixture tightly into a clean glass jar, pressing down firmly to remove any air bubbles.

4.   Pour filtered water over the cabbage until it's completely submerged, leaving about 1 inch of space at the top of the jar.

5.   Place a clean weight or fermentation weight on top of the cabbage to keep it submerged under the water.

6.   Cover the jar with a clean cloth or lid, and let it ferment at room temperature for 1-2 weeks, depending on your taste preference.

7.   Once fermented to your liking, transfer the sauerkraut to the refrigerator to slow down the fermentation process.

8.   Enjoy as a tangy and probiotic-rich addition to meals or snacks.

5. Homemade Nutrient-Packed Trail Mixes

Superfood Trail Mix

- **Ingredients:**

  - 1 cup raw almonds

  - 1 cup raw cashews

  - 1/2 cup pumpkin seeds

  - 1/2 cup dried goji berries

  - 1/2 cup dried cranberries

  - 1/4 cup dark chocolate chips or cacao nibs

  - Optional: unsweetened coconut flakes

- **Instructions:**

1. In a large bowl, combine raw almonds, raw cashews, pumpkin seeds, dried goji berries, dried cranberries, and dark chocolate chips or cacao nibs.

2. Mix well to distribute ingredients evenly.

3.   Store trail mix in an airtight container or portion into individual snack bags for grab-and-go convenience.

4.   Enjoy as a nutrient-packed snack on hikes, road trips, or anytime you need a boost of energy.

Chapter 6:

Desserts

Raw Vegan Brownie Bites

- o **Ingredients:**

  - 1 cup Medjool dates, pitted

  - 1 cup raw walnuts

  - 3 tablespoons unsweetened cocoa powder

  - Pinch of salt

  - Optional toppings: shredded coconut, chopped nuts

- o **Instructions:**

1. Place pitted dates in a food processor and process until they form a sticky paste.

2. Add raw walnuts, unsweetened cocoa powder, and a pinch of salt to the food processor. Process until well combined and the mixture sticks together.

3.   Roll the mixture into small balls and coat with optional toppings like shredded coconut or chopped nuts.

4.   Place the brownie bites in the refrigerator to firm up for at least 30 minutes before serving.

5.   Enjoy these guilt-free indulgent treats!

2. Fruit-Focused Dessert Delights

Baked Cinnamon Apple Slices

- **Ingredients:**
    - 2 large apples, cored and thinly sliced
    - 1 tablespoon maple syrup or honey
    - 1 teaspoon ground cinnamon
    - Pinch of nutmeg
    - Optional toppings: chopped nuts, granola, yogurt
- **Instructions:**

1.   Preheat the oven to 350°F (175°C) and line a baking sheet with parchment paper.

2.   In a bowl, toss apple slices with maple syrup or honey, ground cinnamon, and nutmeg until evenly coated.

3.   Spread the apple slices in a single layer on the prepared baking sheet.

4.   Bake for 20-25 minutes, until apples are tender and lightly caramelized.

5.   Serve baked cinnamon apple slices warm with optional toppings like chopped nuts, granola, or a dollop of yogurt.

3. Decadent Chocolate Creations

Avocado Chocolate Mousse

- o **Ingredients:**

  - 2 ripe avocados
  - 1/4 cup unsweetened cocoa powder

- 1/4 cup maple syrup or honey

- 1 teaspoon vanilla extract

- Pinch of salt

- Optional toppings: shaved chocolate, berries, whipped coconut cream

- **Instructions:**

1. Scoop the flesh of the avocados into a food processor.

2. Add unsweetened cocoa powder, maple syrup or honey, vanilla extract, and a pinch of salt.

3. Blend until smooth and creamy, scraping down the sides of the food processor as needed.

4. Transfer the avocado chocolate mousse to serving bowls or glasses.

5. Chill in the refrigerator for at least 30 minutes before serving.

6. Garnish with optional toppings like shaved chocolate, berries, or whipped coconut cream.

4. Dairy-Free Ice Creams and Sorbets

Coconut Mango Sorbet

- **Ingredients:**

  - 2 cups frozen mango chunks

  - 1/2 cup coconut milk

  - 2 tablespoons maple syrup or honey

  - 1 tablespoon lime juice

  - Zest of 1 lime (optional)

- **Instructions:**

1. In a blender, combine frozen mango chunks, coconut milk, maple syrup or honey, lime juice, and lime zest if using.

2. Blend until smooth and creamy, adding more coconut milk if needed to achieve desired consistency.

3. Transfer the mixture to an ice cream maker and churn according to the manufacturer's instructions until sorbet is thickened.

4.   Serve coconut mango sorbet immediately for a soft-serve texture, or transfer to a container and freeze for a firmer texture.

5.   Enjoy this refreshing dairy-free treat on a hot day!

5. Sweet Bites for Any Occasion

No-Bake Energy Bites

- o **Ingredients:**

  - 1 cup rolled oats

  - 1/2 cup almond butter or peanut butter

  - 1/4 cup honey or maple syrup

  - 1/4 cup shredded coconut

- 1/4 cup mini chocolate chips

- 1 teaspoon vanilla extract

- Pinch of salt

o **Instructions:**

1. In a large bowl, combine rolled oats, almond butter or peanut butter, honey or maple syrup, shredded coconut, mini chocolate chips, vanilla extract, and a pinch of salt.

2. Stir until all ingredients are well combined and form a sticky mixture.

3. Using clean hands, roll the mixture into small balls, about 1 inch in diameter.

4. Place energy bites on a baking sheet lined with parchment paper and refrigerate for at least 30 minutes to firm up.

5. Store energy bites in an airtight container in the refrigerator for up to one week, or freeze for longer storage.

6. Enjoy these sweet and satisfying bites as a quick snack or dessert anytime!

Chapter 7:

Beverages

Hydrating Infusions and Teas

Citrus Mint Infused Water

- Ingredients:

    o 1 lemon, sliced

    o 1 lime, sliced

- o   1 orange, sliced

- o   Handful of fresh mint leaves

- o   Ice cubes

- o   Filtered water

- **How to Make:**

1.   In a pitcher, combine the sliced lemon, lime, and orange.

2.   Add a handful of fresh mint leaves.

3.   Fill the pitcher with filtered water and add ice cubes.

4.   Stir gently to mix the ingredients.

5.   Refrigerate for at least 30 minutes to allow the flavors to infuse.

6.   Serve chilled over ice and enjoy.

- **Nutritional Value (per serving):**

- o   Calories: 10

- o   Carbohydrates: 3g

- o   Sugars: 1g

- ○ Vitamin C: 15% of the Daily Value (DV)

- **Time/Serving:**

  - ○ Prep Time: 10 minutes

  - ○ Infusion Time: 30 minutes

  - ○ Servings: 4

Recipe: Ginger Turmeric Tea

- **Ingredients:**

  - ○ 4 cups water

  - ○ 1-inch piece of fresh ginger, sliced

  - ○ 1 teaspoon ground turmeric (or 1-inch piece fresh turmeric, sliced)

  - ○ 1 tablespoon honey or maple syrup (optional)

  - ○ Juice of 1 lemon

  - ○ Pinch of black pepper

- **How to Make:**

1. In a saucepan, bring 4 cups of water to a boil.

2. Add the sliced ginger and turmeric to the boiling water.

3. Reduce heat and let it simmer for 10-15 minutes.

4. Strain the tea into a teapot or pitcher.

5. Add honey or maple syrup if desired, and stir in the lemon juice and a pinch of black pepper.

6. Serve hot and enjoy.

- **Nutritional Value (per serving):**
  - Calories: 20
  - Carbohydrates: 5g
  - Sugars: 4g
  - Vitamin C: 10% of the DV

- **Time/Serving:**
  - Prep Time: 5 minutes
  - Cook Time: 15 minutes
  - Servings: 4

Recipe: Hibiscus Iced Tea

- **Ingredients:**

  - 4 cups water

  - 1/2 cup dried hibiscus flowers

  - 1-2 tablespoons honey or agave syrup (optional)

  - Juice of 1 lime

  - Ice cubes

  - Fresh mint leaves (optional for garnish)

- **How to Make:**

1. In a saucepan, bring 4 cups of water to a boil.

2. Remove from heat and add the dried hibiscus flowers.

3. Let the hibiscus steep for 10-15 minutes.

4. Strain the tea into a teapot or pitcher.

5. Add honey or agave syrup if desired, and stir in the lime juice.

6.	Let the tea cool to room temperature, then refrigerate until chilled.

7.	Serve over ice and garnish with fresh mint leaves if desired.

- **Nutritional Value (per serving):**

  o Calories: 15

  o Carbohydrates: 4g

  o Sugars: 3g

  o Vitamin C: 5% of the DV

- **Time/Serving:**

  o Prep Time: 5 minutes

  o Steep Time: 15 minutes

  o Chill Time: 30 minutes

  o Servings: 4

Recipe: Green Goddess Smoothie

- **Ingredients:**

- o   1 cup spinach leaves

- o   1/2 ripe avocado

- o   1/2 cup frozen pineapple chunks

- o   1/2 cup coconut water

- o   1 tablespoon chia seeds

- o   Optional: 1 scoop of protein powder

- **How to Make:**

1.   Add all ingredients to a blender.

2.   Blend until smooth and creamy.

3.   Pour into a glass and enjoy immediately.

- **Nutritional Value (per serving):**

- o   Calories: 150

- o   Carbohydrates: 20g

- o   Protein: 3g

- o   Fat: 8g

- o   Fiber: 6g

- o   Vitamin C: 70% of the DV

- **Time/Serving:**

  - Prep Time: 5 minutes

  - Servings: 1

Recipe: Carrot Ginger Juice

- **Ingredients:**

  - 4 large carrots, peeled

  - 1-inch piece of fresh ginger

  - 1 apple, cored

  - 1 tablespoon lemon juice

  - Water (if needed for consistency)

- **How to Make:**

1. Run the carrots, ginger, and apple through a juicer.

2. Stir in the lemon juice.

3. Add water if needed to adjust the consistency.

4. Serve over ice if desired and enjoy.

- **Nutritional Value (per serving):**

  - Calories: 90

  - Carbohydrates: 22g

  - Sugars: 15g

  - Fiber: 3g

  - Vitamin A: 380% of the DV

  - Vitamin C: 30% of the DV

- **Time/Serving:**

  - Prep Time: 10 minutes

  - Servings: 2

Recipe: Blueberry Banana Smoothie

- **Ingredients:**

  - 1 cup frozen blueberries

  - 1 ripe banana

  - 1 cup almond milk (or other non-dairy milk)

- o   1 tablespoon almond butter

- o   1 teaspoon honey or maple syrup (optional)

- **How to Make:**

1. Add all ingredients to a blender.

2. Blend until smooth and creamy.

3. Pour into a glass and enjoy immediately.

- **Nutritional Value (per serving):**

  - o   Calories: 200

  - o   Carbohydrates: 36g

  - o   Protein: 4g

  - o   Fat: 6g

  - o   Fiber: 6g

  - o   Vitamin C: 25% of the DV

- **Time/Serving:**

  - o   Prep Time: 5 minutes

  - o   Servings: 1

Homemade Nut Milks and Non-Dairy Lattes

Recipe: Almond Milk

- **Ingredients:**

    o 1 cup raw almonds, soaked overnight

    o 4 cups filtered water

    o 1-2 dates, pitted (optional for sweetness)

    o 1 teaspoon vanilla extract (optional)

    o Pinch of salt

- **How to Make:**

1. Drain and rinse soaked almonds.

2. In a blender, combine soaked almonds and filtered water.

3. Blend on high speed for 1-2 minutes until smooth and creamy.

4. Strain the almond mixture through a nut milk bag or fine mesh strainer into a large bowl or pitcher.

5.   Rinse out the blender and return the strained almond milk.

6.   Add dates, vanilla extract, and a pinch of salt (if using) to the almond milk and blend until smooth.

7.   Store almond milk in a sealed container in the refrigerator for up to 5 days.

8.   Enjoy homemade almond milk in lattes, smoothies, or over cereal.

- **Nutritional Value (per serving):**

    o   Calories: 40

    o   Carbohydrates: 2g

    o   Protein: 1g

    o   Fat: 3.5g

    o   Calcium: 2% of the DV

- **Time/Serving:**

    o   Prep Time: 10 minutes (plus soaking time)

    o   Servings: 4

Recipe: Cashew Milk

- **Ingredients:**

  - 1 cup raw cashews, soaked for 2-4 hours

  - 4 cups filtered water

  - 1-2 dates, pitted (optional for sweetness)

  - 1 teaspoon vanilla extract (optional)

  - Pinch of salt

- **How to Make:**

1. Drain and rinse soaked cashews.

2. In a blender, combine soaked cashews and filtered water.

3. Blend on high speed for 1-2 minutes until smooth and creamy.

4. Strain the cashew mixture through a nut milk bag or fine mesh strainer into a large bowl or pitcher.

5. Rinse out the blender and return the strained cashew milk.

6.   Add dates, vanilla extract, and a pinch of salt (if using) to the cashew milk and blend until smooth.

7.   Store cashew milk in a sealed container in the refrigerator for up to 5 days.

8.   Enjoy homemade cashew milk in lattes, smoothies, or over cereal.

- **Nutritional Value (per serving):**

  - Calories: 50

  - Carbohydrates: 3g

  - Protein: 1g

  - Fat: 4g

  - Calcium: 2% of the DV

- **Time/Serving:**

  - Prep Time: 10 minutes (plus soaking time)

  - Servings: 4

Recipe: Golden Turmeric Latte

- **Ingredients:**

  - 2 cups almond milk (or other non-dairy milk)

  - 1 teaspoon ground turmeric

  - 1/2 teaspoon ground cinnamon

  - 1/4 teaspoon ground ginger

  - 1 tablespoon honey or maple syrup (optional)

  - Pinch of black pepper

- **How to Make:**

1. In a small saucepan, heat the almond milk over medium heat until warm.

2. Add ground turmeric, ground cinnamon, ground ginger, honey or maple syrup (if using), and a pinch of black pepper.

3. Whisk continuously until the mixture is hot and well combined.

4. Pour the latte into mugs.

5.   Serve immediately and enjoy.

- **Nutritional Value (per serving):**

  - Calories: 80

  - Carbohydrates: 12g

  - Protein: 1g

  - Fat: 3g

  - Calcium: 20% of the DV

- **Time/Serving:**

  - Prep Time: 5 minutes

Chapter 8:

Condiments and Sauces

1. Homemade Salad Dressings and Vinaigrettes

Classic Vinaigrette

- **Ingredients:**

    o   3 tablespoons extra-virgin olive oil

    o   1 tablespoon red wine vinegar

    o   1 teaspoon Dijon mustard

    o   1 small garlic clove, minced

    o   Salt and pepper to taste

- **Instructions:**

1.   Whisk together vinegar, mustard, and garlic.

2.   Slowly drizzle in olive oil while whisking until emulsified.

3.   Season with salt and pepper.

- **Nutritional Info (per serving, 2 tablespoons):**

- o Calories: 140

- o Fat: 14g

- o Carbohydrates: 1g

- o Protein: 0g

- **Time:**

  - o Prep: 5 minutes

  - o Total: 5 minutes

Creamy Caesar Dressing

- **Ingredients:**

  - o 1 cup mayonnaise

  - o 1/2 cup grated Parmesan cheese

  - o 2 tablespoons lemon juice

  - o 1 tablespoon Dijon mustard

  - o 2 teaspoons Worcestershire sauce

  - o 2 garlic cloves, minced

  - o Salt and pepper to taste

- **Instructions:**

1. Combine all ingredients in a bowl.

2. Whisk until smooth.

3. Adjust seasoning with salt and pepper.

- **Nutritional Info (per serving, 2 tablespoons):**

  o Calories: 180

  o Fat: 18g

  o Carbohydrates: 2g

  o Protein: 2g

- **Time:**

  o Prep: 5 minutes

  o Total: 5 minutes

2. Flavorful Marinades and Rubs

Lemon Herb Marinade

- **Ingredients:**

  o 1/4 cup olive oil

  o 1/4 cup lemon juice

  o 2 garlic cloves, minced

- o 1 tablespoon chopped fresh rosemary

- o 1 tablespoon chopped fresh thyme

- o Salt and pepper to taste

- **Instructions:**

1. Mix all ingredients in a bowl.

2. Marinate meat for at least 30 minutes.

- **Nutritional Info (per serving, 2 tablespoons):**

  - o Calories: 120

  - o Fat: 13g

  - o Carbohydrates: 2g

  - o Protein: 0g

- **Time:**

  - o Prep: 5 minutes

  - o Marinate: 30 minutes

  - o Total: 35 minutes

BBQ Spice Rub

- **Ingredients:**

    o 2 tablespoons brown sugar

    o 1 tablespoon smoked paprika

    o 1 tablespoon garlic powder

    o 1 tablespoon onion powder

    o 1 teaspoon black pepper

    o 1 teaspoon salt

    o 1 teaspoon cayenne pepper

- **Instructions:**

1. Combine all ingredients in a bowl.

2. Rub evenly over meat before grilling or baking.

- **Nutritional Info (per serving, 1 tablespoon):**

    o Calories: 25

    o Fat: 0g

    o Carbohydrates: 6g

    o Protein: 0g

- **Time:**

  - Prep: 5 minutes

  - Total: 5 minutes

---

3. Dipping Sauces and Spreads

Spicy Sriracha Mayo

- **Ingredients:**

  - 1/2 cup mayonnaise

  - 2 tablespoons Sriracha sauce

  - 1 teaspoon lime juice

  - Pinch of salt

- **Instructions:**

1. Mix all ingredients in a bowl.

2. Serve as a dipping sauce or spread.

- **Nutritional Info (per serving, 2 tablespoons):**

  - Calories: 140

  - Fat: 15g

  - Carbohydrates: 1g

- o Protein: 0g

- **Time:**

  - o Prep: 5 minutes

  - o Total: 5 minutes

Classic Hummus

- **Ingredients:**

  - o 1 can (15 oz) chickpeas, drained

  - o 1/4 cup tahini

  - o 2 tablespoons olive oil

  - o 2 tablespoons lemon juice

  - o 2 garlic cloves, minced

  - o Salt to taste

- **Instructions:**

1. Combine all ingredients in a food processor.

2. Blend until smooth.

3. Adjust seasoning with salt and more lemon juice if needed.

- **Nutritional Info (per serving, 2 tablespoons):**

  - Calories: 70

  - Fat: 4g

  - Carbohydrates: 6g

  - Protein: 2g

- **Time:**

  - Prep: 10 minutes

  - Total: 10 minutes

4. Gut-Healing Broths and Stocks

Bone Broth

- **Ingredients:**

  - 2 lbs beef or chicken bones

  - 1 onion, quartered

  - 2 carrots, chopped

  - 2 celery stalks, chopped

  - 2 tablespoons apple cider vinegar

  - 10 cups water

- o   Salt and pepper to taste

- **Instructions:**

1. Combine all ingredients in a large pot.

2. Bring to a boil, then simmer for 12-24 hours.

3. Strain the broth and season with salt and pepper.

- **Nutritional Info (per serving, 1 cup):**

  - o   Calories: 50

  - o   Fat: 2g

  - o   Carbohydrates: 2g

  - o   Protein: 5g

- **Time:**

  - o   Prep: 10 minutes

  - o   Cook: 12-24 hours

  - o   Total: 12-24 hours 10 minutes

Vegetable Stock

- **Ingredients:**

  - 1 onion, chopped

  - 2 carrots, chopped

  - 2 celery stalks, chopped

  - 1 garlic clove, minced

  - 1 bay leaf

  - 10 cups water

  - Salt and pepper to taste

- **Instructions:**

1. Combine all ingredients in a large pot.

2. Bring to a boil, then simmer for 1-2 hours.

3. Strain the stock and season with salt and pepper.

- **Nutritional Info (per serving, 1 cup):**

  - Calories: 10

  - Fat: 0g

- o Carbohydrates: 2g

- o Protein: 0g

- **Time:**

  - o Prep: 10 minutes

  - o Cook: 1-2 hours

  - o Total: 1-2 hours 10 minutes

5. Essential DIY Seasoning Blends

Italian Seasoning

- **Ingredients:**

  - o 2 tablespoons dried basil

  - o 2 tablespoons dried oregano

  - o 1 tablespoon dried rosemary

  - o 1 tablespoon dried thyme

  - o 1 tablespoon dried marjoram

  - o 1 teaspoon garlic powder

- **Instructions:**

1. Combine all ingredients in a bowl.

2. Store in an airtight container.

- **Nutritional Info (per serving, 1 teaspoon):**

  - Calories: 5

  - Fat: 0g

  - Carbohydrates: 1g

  - Protein: 0g

- **Time:**

  - Prep: 5 minutes

  - Total: 5 minutes

Taco Seasoning

- **Ingredients:**

  - 1 tablespoon chili powder

  - 1 teaspoon garlic powder

  - 1 teaspoon onion powder

  - 1 teaspoon paprika

  - 1 teaspoon ground cumin

  - 1/2 teaspoon oregano

- 1/2 teaspoon salt

- 1/2 teaspoon black pepper

- **Instructions:**

1. Combine all ingredients in a bowl.

2. Store in an airtight container.

- **Nutritional Info (per serving, 1 teaspoon):**

  - Calories: 5

  - Fat: 0g

  - Carbohydrates: 1g

  - Protein: 0g

- **Time:**

  - Prep: 5 minutes

  - Total: 5 minutes

Chapter 9:

Special Occasion Menus

Roast Turkey with Herb Butter

- **Ingredients:**

    o   1 whole turkey (12-14 lbs)

    o   1/2 cup unsalted butter, softened

    o   1/4 cup chopped fresh herbs (rosemary, thyme, sage)

    o   2 garlic cloves, minced

    o   Salt and pepper to taste

- **Instructions:**

1.   Preheat oven to 325°F (165°C).

2.   Mix butter, herbs, garlic, salt, and pepper.

3.   Rub mixture under the turkey's skin and over the surface.

4.   Roast turkey in the oven for 3-4 hours, basting occasionally.

5.   Let rest for 20 minutes before carving.

- **Nutritional Info (per serving, 6 oz turkey):**

  o   Calories: 340

  o   Fat: 20g

  o   Carbohydrates: 0g

  o   Protein: 40g

- **Time:**

  o   Prep: 30 minutes

  o   Cook: 3-4 hours

  o   Total: 3.5-4.5 hours

Classic Mashed Potatoes

- **Ingredients:**

  o   3 lbs potatoes, peeled and cubed

  o   1/2 cup unsalted butter

  o   1 cup whole milk

- o   Salt and pepper to taste

- **Instructions:**

1. Boil potatoes until tender, about 20 minutes.

2. Drain and mash potatoes.

3. Add butter, milk, salt, and pepper. Mix until smooth.

- **Nutritional Info (per serving, 1 cup):**

  - o   Calories: 200

  - o   Fat: 10g

  - o   Carbohydrates: 25g

  - o   Protein: 4g

- **Time:**

  - o   Prep: 10 minutes

  - o   Cook: 20 minutes

  - o   Total: 30 minutes

Beef Wellington

- **Ingredients:**

  - 1.5 lbs beef tenderloin

  - 2 tablespoons olive oil

  - 1/2 lb mushrooms, finely chopped

  - 1 shallot, minced

  - 2 tablespoons Dijon mustard

  - 4 slices prosciutto

  - 1 sheet puff pastry

  - 1 egg, beaten

  - Salt and pepper to taste

- **Instructions:**

1. Preheat oven to 400°F (200°C).

2. Sear beef in oil, season with salt and pepper. Let cool.

3.   Cook mushrooms and shallot until moisture evaporates.

4.   Spread mustard over beef, wrap with prosciutto and mushroom mixture.

5.   Wrap in puff pastry, brush with beaten egg.

6.   Bake for 25-30 minutes until golden.

- **Nutritional Info (per serving, 6 oz):**
  - Calories: 560
  - Fat: 36g
  - Carbohydrates: 24g
  - Protein: 36g
- **Time:**
  - Prep: 30 minutes
  - Cook: 30 minutes
  - Total: 1 hour

Roasted Asparagus with Lemon

- **Ingredients:**

- o 1 lb asparagus, trimmed

- o 2 tablespoons olive oil

- o 1 lemon, zested and juiced

- o Salt and pepper to taste

- **Instructions:**

1. Preheat oven to 425°F (220°C).

2. Toss asparagus with olive oil, lemon zest, and juice.

3. Season with salt and pepper.

4. Roast for 12-15 minutes until tender.

- **Nutritional Info (per serving, 1/2 cup):**

- o Calories: 60

- o Fat: 4g

- o Carbohydrates: 6g

- o Protein: 2g

- **Time:**

- o Prep: 5 minutes

- o Cook: 15 minutes

- o Total: 20 minutes

---

3. Seasonal Gathering Ideas

Pumpkin Soup

- **Ingredients:**

  - o 2 tablespoons olive oil

  - o 1 onion, chopped

  - o 2 garlic cloves, minced

  - o 4 cups pumpkin puree

  - o 4 cups vegetable broth

  - o 1 cup heavy cream

  - o Salt, pepper, and nutmeg to taste

- **Instructions:**

1. Heat oil, sauté onion and garlic until soft.

2. Add pumpkin puree and broth, bring to a simmer.

3.   Stir in cream, season with salt, pepper, and nutmeg.

4.   Simmer for 10 minutes.

- **Nutritional Info (per serving, 1 cup):**

  o Calories: 180

  o Fat: 14g

  o Carbohydrates: 15g

  o Protein: 3g

- **Time:**

  o Prep: 10 minutes

  o Cook: 20 minutes

  o Total: 30 minutes

CONCLUSION

In creating meals for various occasions—from holiday feasts to stylish dinner parties, seasonal gatherings, healthy picnics, and private date nights—the culinary journey intertwines with the art of food, celebration, and connection. Each recipe represents not just flavors, but also memories, traditions, and the spirit of togetherness.

As we enter into the world of holiday feasts, the famous roast turkey with herb butter evokes images of busy kitchens, families gathering around tables filled with warmth and abundance. Paired with creamy mashed potatoes, it forms the cornerstone of beloved customs, while its succulence and aromatic herbs excite the senses, creating a medley of flavors that stay long after the last bite.

Transitioning to elegant dinner parties, the Beef Wellington emerges as the epitome of culinary grace, representing class and culinary skill. Wrapped in layers of prosciutto and puff pastry, the soft beef tenderloin becomes a culinary creation, asking guests to enjoy every decadent bite. Complemented by roasted asparagus with lemon, the meal strikes a perfect balance between richness and freshness, taking the eating experience to new heights of refinement.

Seasonal parties offer a chance to welcome the gifts of nature, with recipes that celebrate the lively tastes of the season. A creamy pumpkin soup, filled with aromatic spices, brings warmth and comfort, while a cozy apple crisp, adorned with a golden crust of oats and cinnamon, pays homage to the crisp fall air and the fields laden with fruit.

For those wanting healthful food for outdoor activities, healthy picnic and party meals provide a delightful array of choices. From bright salads dressed in homemade vinaigrettes to filling wraps filled with healthy ingredients, these recipes offer a balance of nutrition and taste, perfect for al fresco eating with loved ones.

Lastly, private date nights call for foods that evoke romance and closeness, where every bite becomes a shared moment of connection. Whether it's indulging in a sumptuous plate of spaghetti carbonara or enjoying the delicate flavors of seared scallops with rice, these recipes are meant to spark the senses and create lasting memories.

In conclusion, the art of cooking goes far beyond the world of sustenance—it is a trip of creation, discovery, and joy. Through thoughtfully created meals and recipes, we have the power to feed not only the body but also the mind, encouraging moments of joy, connection, and shared experiences that improve our lives in countless ways. So let us continue to gather around the table, enjoying each dish with thanks and respect for the simple joys that connect us all.

THANKS

READER

www.ingramcontent.com/pod-product-compliance
Lightning Source LLC
Chambersburg PA
CBHW051826250726
48659CB00005B/1691